IMAGINATIONS
Fun Relaxation Stories and Meditations for Kids

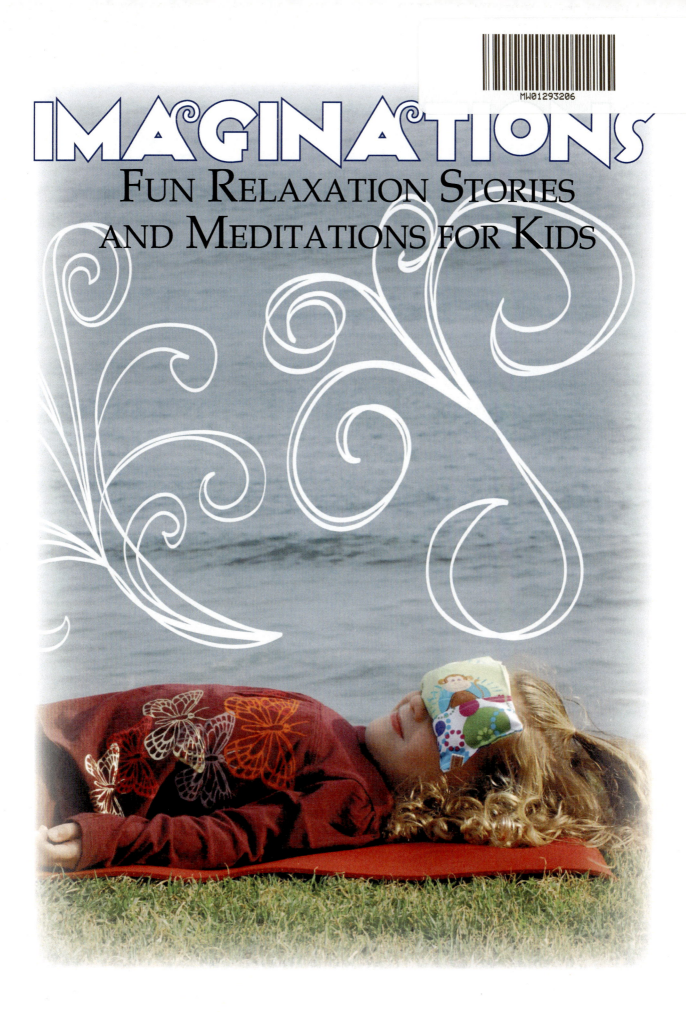

Copyright © 2011 Carolyn Clarke
All rights reserved.

ISBN: 1463512023
ISBN 13: 9781463512026
LCCN: 2011908702
CreateSpace, Charleston, South Carolina

Imaginations

*Fun Relaxation Stories
and Meditations for Kids*

By Carolyn Clarke

Foreword by Laurie Clarke

This book is dedicated to all of the children
in my yoga classes.
Thank you for your joy and laughter.
Thank you for your peace and relaxation.
Namasté. (The light in me sees the light in you.)

Contents

Foreword by Laurie Clarke 5

Introduction for Adults 6

Introduction for Kids 9

Yoga Prep Poses 10

Getting Comfortable 13

Relaxation Stories

    1. A Day at the Beach 16
    2. The Night Sky 18
    3. A Hot Air Balloon Trip 20
    4. Your Bubble 22
    5. Making Friends with a Tree 24
    6. If I Could Fly 26
    7. Clouds in the Sky 28
    8. A Trip in Your Spaceship 30
    9. Enchanted Forest 32
    10. Take a Hike 34
    11. The Love Balloon 36
    12. Under the Sea 38
    13. My Tree House 40
    14. Magic Flower Potion 42
    15. Planting a Seed 44
    16. Finger Lights 46
    17. Loving Kindness 48

Additional Information 50

Acknowledgments

Andrew Beling, my husband and muse. Thank you for being supportive and enthusiastic about this book from the beginning and helping me every step along the way.

Laurie Clarke, my mother. Thank you for showing me the path to relaxation and living by example. Your light continues to shine bright.

Tim Clarke, my dad. Thank you for telling me to take a leap. You were right, the net appeared.

Russell Clarke, my brother. Thank you for filling the world with music and showing me how to follow my creative dreams.

Marsha Wenig and the YogaKids family, Jodi Komitor, Erich Schiffmann, Ti Harmony, Nischala Joy Devi, Ann West and all the yoga teachers with whom I have crossed paths. Thank you for teaching me and inspiring me with ideas, experience, and encouragement.

The Wednesday Supper Club, thank you for keeping my heart light and my belly full.

Megan Crowley, thank you for taking such great photos.

Rory Eslinger, thank you for your beautiful smiles and yoga poses.

And thank you to everyone who read and re-read this book with feedback and encouragement.

Foreword by Laurie Clarke

I have been teaching yoga since 1977. In the beginning I frequently had to explain the difference between yoga and yogurt. Times have definitely changed. Now millions are practicing (and probably eating yogurt, too), and the numbers continue to grow. People are seeking ways to enhance the quality of their existence, to find an oasis in their hectic lives. A guided relaxation offers this refuge where the ever-active mind begins to slow down. We settle into a state of peacefulness, providing the body with the deep rest that it craves. Once students experience how much better they feel, many times after the first class, they will say, "I wish I had found this years ago. I wish I had started when I was young."

As parents and teachers we are always hoping that the guidance we provide our children will help them to lead fulfilled and happy lives. How blessed I felt when my daughter, Carolyn Clarke, joined me in my life's work, adapting it to her own special talents. This book provides you with a lovingly crafted tool to help calm the lively minds of children so they can connect with their own sense of inner peace. What greater gift can we give our children than to plant the seeds of tranquility in their fertile minds?

Love and Namasté,

Laurie Clarke

An Introduction for Adults

The ability to relax is an essential skill in our hectic world today. Kids are shuttled from home to school to afterschool activities and back, often without transition time or down time. We hope that children can lead happy, relaxed, and calm lives, but often we neither teach them how to do this nor do we lead by example. This book provides stories to help children learn to calm their bodies and relax their minds.

The Benefits of Relaxation

Relaxing has many health benefits, including a reduction in stress, a lowering of heart rate, a release of muscle tension, and an overall relaxation response in the body. Relaxation and a child's ability to consciously relax the body and clear the mind can also help address issues such as:

- Anxiety, stress, and excessive worry
- Sleep disorders and nightmares
- Anger issues
- Focus and concentration issues
- Special needs, including ADD, ADHD, Aspergers, autism, OCD
- Depression
- Low self-esteem or negativity
- Grief
- Life changes, such as a move, divorce, change in school, etc.

Relaxation can also address everyday challenges in children's lives. Some examples include:

- Being scared of the dark at bedtime
- Having a bad day at school
- Anxiety about an upcoming test
- Missing a parent who is at work or travelling
- Feeling frustrated over a homework assignment

How to Use This Book

This book is intended as a tool for you to use with your own children or the children you work with as an educator, yoga teacher, therapist, or any other profession involving kids. Use this book when you feel a child needs help bringing his or her energy level down and focusing the mind. Read the relaxation stories, and if you wish, allow the children to complete the activities that can be found on www.ImaginationsForKids.com.

Each relaxation story contains guided imagery for children to imagine. By closing their eyes and imagining what you read, they have the opportunity to relax their bodies and guide their minds.

The stories within this book can be used anytime a child needs to relax. Parents can use them to help children settle down for bed. Teachers can use them as transitions and before tests or activities that require focus and concentration. If there isn't space in a classroom for the children to lie down, have them put their heads down on their desks while you read a relaxation story. If space allows, a relaxation area with cushions or yoga mats can make relaxing even more inviting.

To encourage relaxation, experiment with props or aromatherapy. For example, a spray of lavender oil into the room or a dab smudged in between the eyebrows can help children relax. Try placing an eye pillow filled with flax seeds and herbs over their eyes to help them tune in. A foot massage with lotion will help children wind down. A favorite blanket or pillow can also make the experience more cozy and relaxing.

I have created these relaxation stories for my yoga classes for children. At the end of the class, the children lie down and close their eyes as I talk them through relaxing their bodies (see the section of this book called "Getting Comfortable"). While their bodies are relaxing, I talk them through a relaxation story for their minds to imagine. I have been told by kids time and time again that their favorite part of the yoga class was "the lying down part."

Please keep in mind that these relaxation stories are written in a conversational way, based on how I have said them while teaching. Don't be afraid to improvise with the verbiage, changing the wording so that it flows naturally for you. Try to read the story slowly and in a soothing, calm voice. After reading a story, pause and allow the children to linger in relaxation for as long as they are comfortable. Softly ring a bell or use a calm voice to gently let them know that the story is over if time is an issue. If you are reading the story at bedtime, let your child fall asleep while relaxing.

My hope is that this book brings peacefulness, happiness, and a sense of calm to the children in your lives.

Carolyn Clarke

Introduction for Kids

Adults: Read this to the children in your life.

Yipee! It's time to relax.

Have you had a long day at school, and need a little down time? Are you feeling cranky, worried, or sad about something that happened today? Or, do you feel good, and you want to feel even better?

Relaxing our bodies and focusing our minds helps us to feel happy and healthy. Have fun imagining the stories in this book! Each one is a relaxing adventure and can take you to magical places. You'll have a chance to:

- Play with fairies and gnomes!
- Float in a hot air balloon!
- Swim underwater!
- Go to the beach!
- Build a treehouse!
- And even take a trip in a spaceship!

Ask an adult or friend to read a story to you, and enjoy feeling peaceful and calm.

Have fun and happy relaxing!

Carolyn

Yoga Prep Poses

Adults: Yoga can be used as a way to prepare children for relaxation. These are the poses that I use in my yoga classes to transition from activity to relaxation. There are many reasons for this, primarily that lying on the back helps the body relax. This position actually activates the part of the nervous system that is responsible for the relaxation response in the body (the parasympathetic nervous system). Another reason is that the child is grounded in one place instead of roaming around. Also, there is less distraction lying on the ground, because your eyes naturally go to the ceiling instead of around the room.

Here are some fun yoga poses that can be done before any relaxation story in this book:

Knee Hug

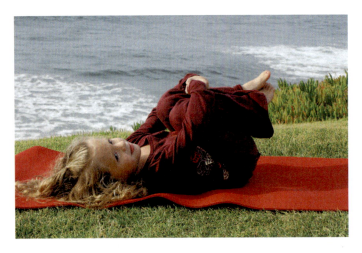

1. Lie down on the ground or bed.
2. Bring your knees to your chest.
3. Wrap your arms around your knees like you are giving yourself a big hug.

Happy Baby

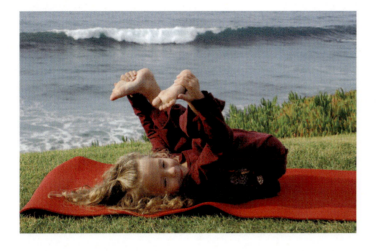

1. From Knee Hug, let go of your legs with your arms.
2. Keep your knees bent, and reach your feet up in the air.
3. Reach with your arms for your feet.

Legs Up

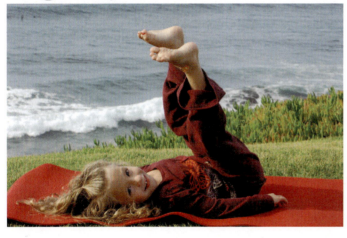

1. From Happy Baby, let go of your feet.
2. Reach your legs straight up in the air.
3. This pose can also be done with your legs resting on a wall.

Starfish (or "Savasana")

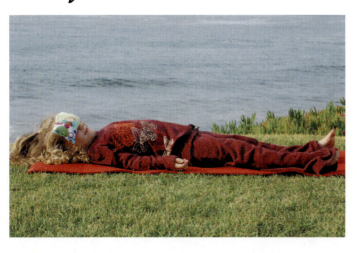

1. From Legs Up, bring your legs down one at a time.
2. Stretch your legs out on the ground with a little space between your feet.
3. Lay your arms along the sides of your body, palms up to the sky.

Note: Starfish Pose, or Savasana, can be used for any of the following stories.

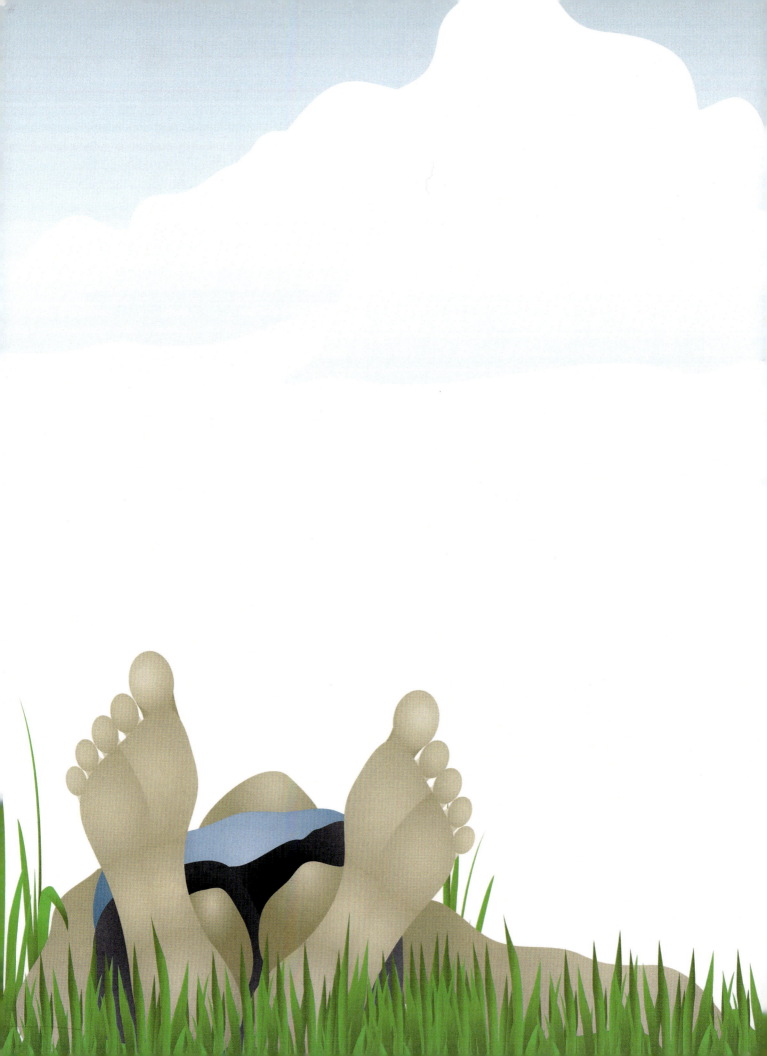

Getting Comfortable

Adults: Try starting each story by having the children settle their bodies and "Get Comfortable."

Are you comfortable?
Well, try this:
Lie down in Starfish Pose.
Squeeze your toe muscles gently, and then let them relax.
Now squeeze your legs all the way down to your toes, tight, tight, tight…
And let them relax.
Now squeeze your belly gently, and then let it go.
Now squeeze all the muscles in your arms and hands.
Make a fist, squeeze it tight, and then let your arms relax and flop down to the ground.
Now squeeze all the muscles in your face, like a raisin face, and then let them relax to make a smooth face.
Now feel your whole body melting into the ground, like ice cream on a hot summer day.
Feel loose and limp like a cooked noodle.
Feel how relaxed and calm your body is.
Now you are comfortable!

Note: This exercise can be done alone or before another relaxation story. You can say:
"While your body is relaxing, here is a story for you to imagine." Choose any of the relaxation stories on the following pages.

Relaxation

Stories

A Day at the Beach

Imagine you are walking on the beach.

Feel the sand between your toes. Is it wet or dry?

When you find your perfect spot,

Spread out your towel and lie down in the sand.

Feel the warm sun on your skin and a cool, refreshing breeze.

Listen to the waves crashing on the shore…

Children playing…

Seagulls singing…

And people laughing.

Listen to the sound of the waves.

A wave comes into shore, and then the wave moves back into the ocean.

Now, put your hand on your belly.

Feel it rise up when you take in a breath,

And feel it fall down when you let out a breath.

Up and down, in and out. Just like the waves in the ocean…

Enjoy lying here feeling your body relaxed at the beach.

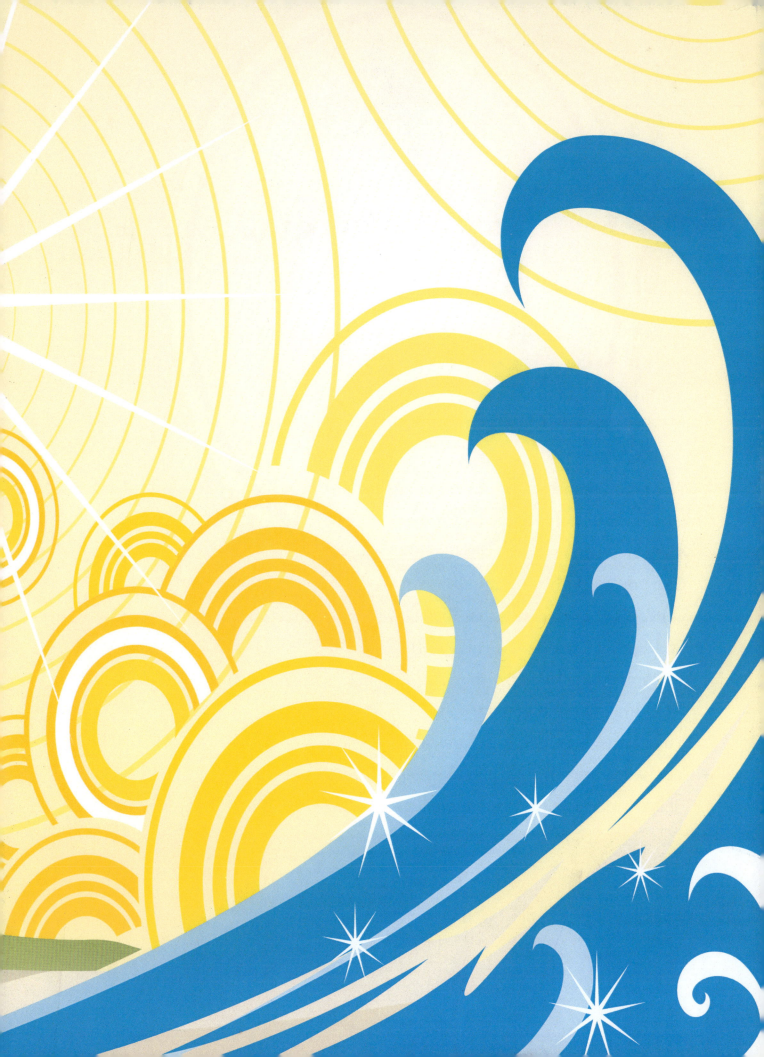

The Night Sky

Imagine you are lying in your bed at night.

Look up at the ceiling,

And imagine the roof opens up so you can see the night sky.

An owl flies above you—

"Who?" "Who?"

The moon shines into your room and makes everything glow.

Up above you is a sky full of stars.

They twinkle and shimmer like diamonds.

Can you count how many there are?

Do you see any shapes that the stars make or constellations?

Suddenly you see a shooting star!

You must be very lucky to see one, so make a wish!

Now imagine that you are a star.

Your arms, legs, and head are each a point of the star.

You shine and twinkle just like a star in the sky.

Relax and know that you are just as brilliant as the stars in the sky.

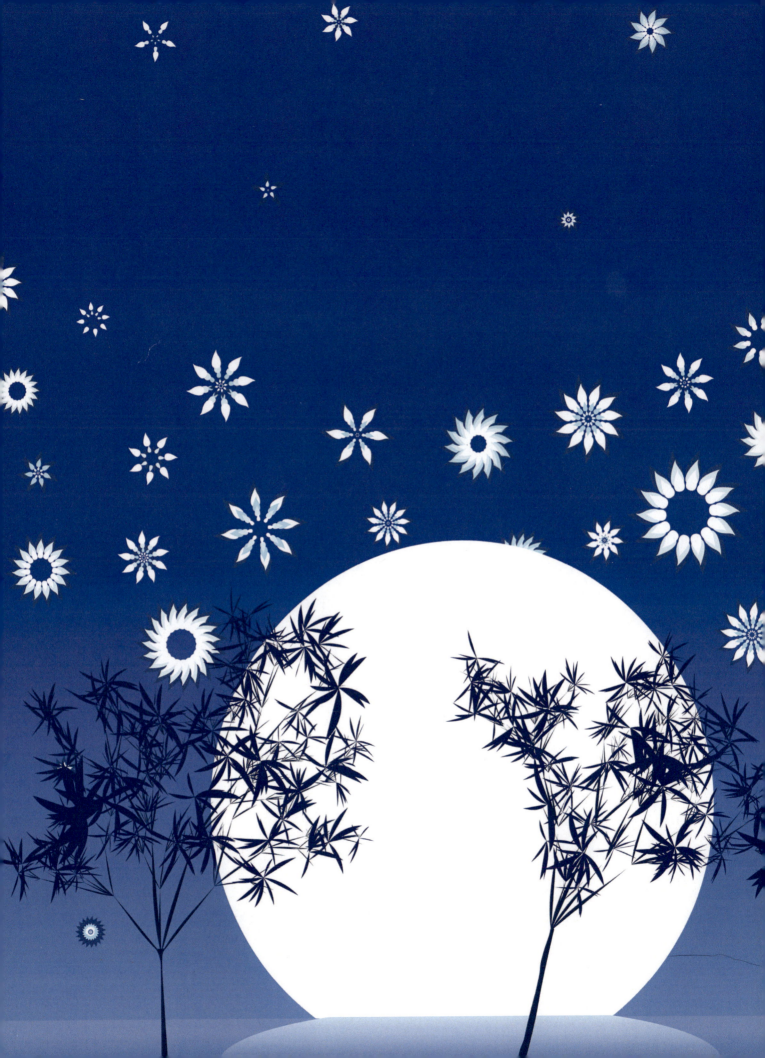

A Hot Air Balloon Trip

Imagine you climb into a great big hot air balloon.

What color is your balloon?

Your favorite color?

All the colors of the rainbow?

Polka dotted?

Take in a big breath, and then blow out, filling up your hot air balloon.

Feel your hot air balloon lift up off the ground and float into the sky.

Do you see any birds, planes, or clouds?

Look down—I think you are flying over your house!

Now choose where you are going to fly, anywhere you want to go.

The beach…the mountains…the North Pole…the desert…the jungle…

Once you get there, feel your balloon land gently.

Imagine you climb out of your balloon to explore.

What do you see?

What do you smell?

What do you hear?

What do you feel?

Do you taste anything?

Now climb back into your balloon.

Wave goodbye to any friends you have made.

Take in a big breath and then blow out, filling up your hot air balloon again.

Feel it lift up off the ground and float back home.

Land your hot air balloon on the ground, safe and sound.

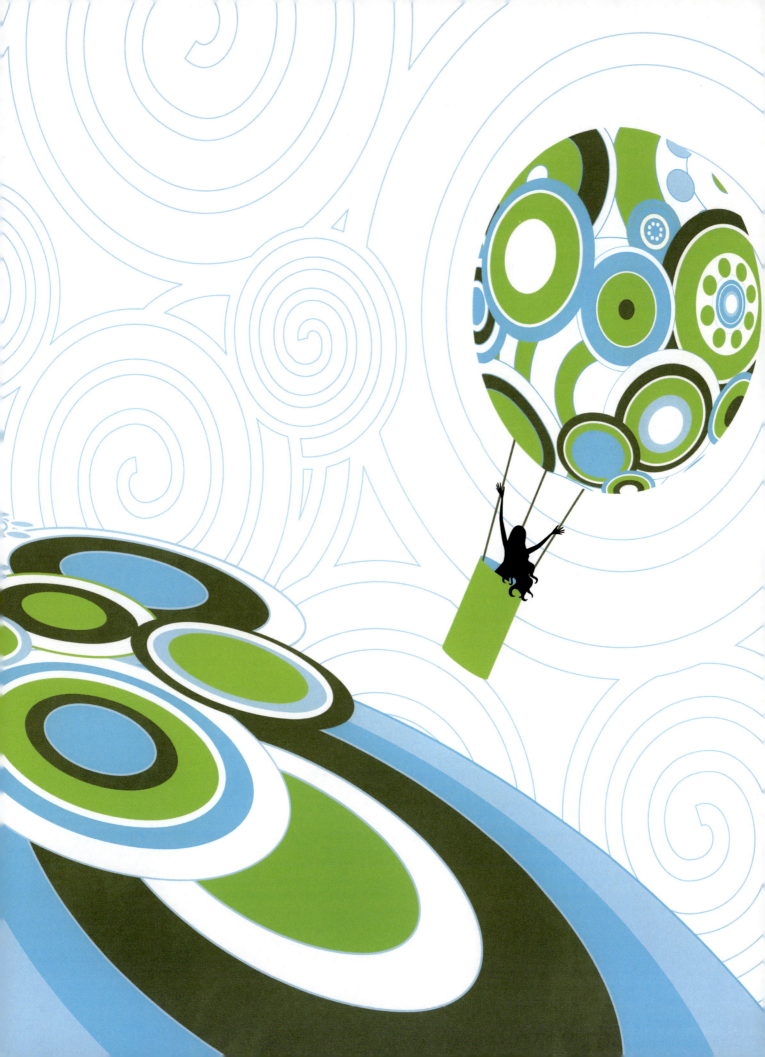

Your Bubble

Imagine you have a bottle of bubble soap.

Open the lid.

Take out the magic bubble wand.

Now imagine that you blow a bubble.

It gets bigger and bigger and bigger…

It's as big as your head now.

And then it gets bigger…

And bigger…

And bigger.

It is so big that it gently wraps around you.

What color is your bubble?

Is there anything or anyone inside your bubble with you?

What sounds do you hear?

What does it smell like?

Feel how safe you are inside your very own bubble world.

Nothing can hurt you here.

When you are ready, imagine that you take your finger and gently poke at the bubble until it pops.

The air slowly leaves the bubble, and you begin to see the room around you.

Anytime you are scared, just imagine yourself in your own safe bubble.

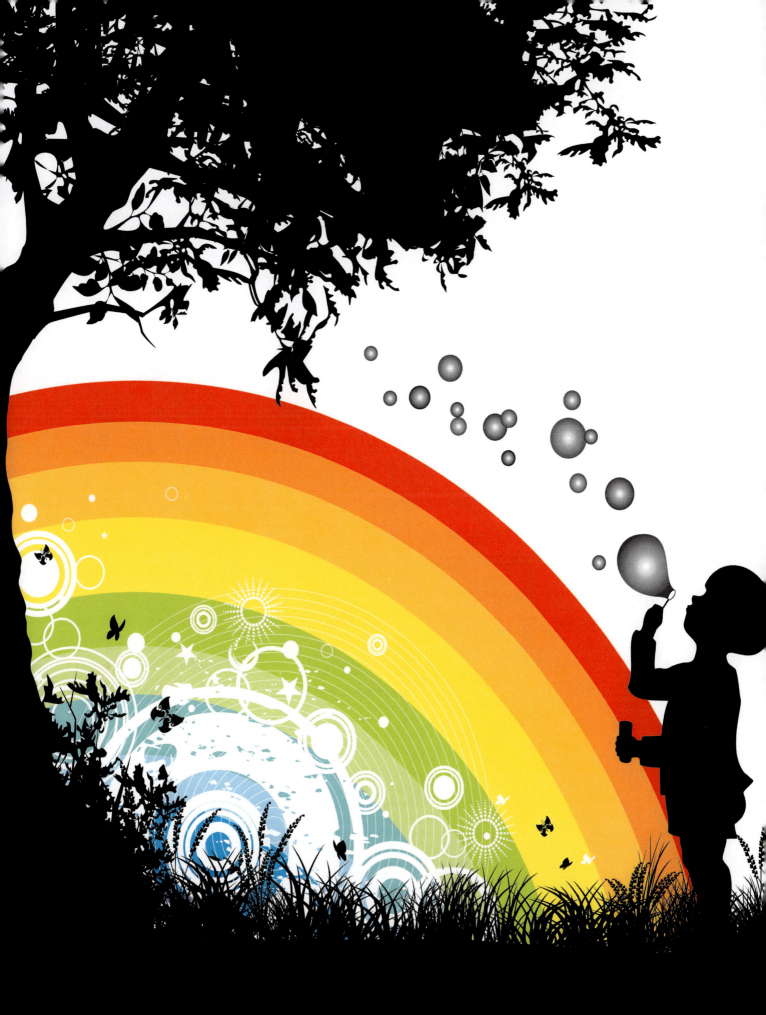

Making Friends with a Tree

Imagine that you are walking through a forest.

Any tree you can imagine is here in this forest.

Apple trees, maple trees, palm trees…

Sycamore trees, banana trees, orange trees…

Even imaginary trees are here in this forest, like candy trees and trees that grant wishes.

Imagine walking over to any tree that you like.

Touch its bark and notice how it feels on your skin.

Sniff its leaves.

If it has fruit, take a bite and see what it tastes like.

Now imagine you climb its branches, feeling very safe.

When you reach the top, look out and see all of the trees in this forest.

Now climb back down and take a rest in your tree's shade.

Take some time to enjoy being with your new tree buddy.

Trees breathe out what we breathe in.

So, take a deep breath full of oxygen,

And then slowly let it out so the tree can breathe, too.

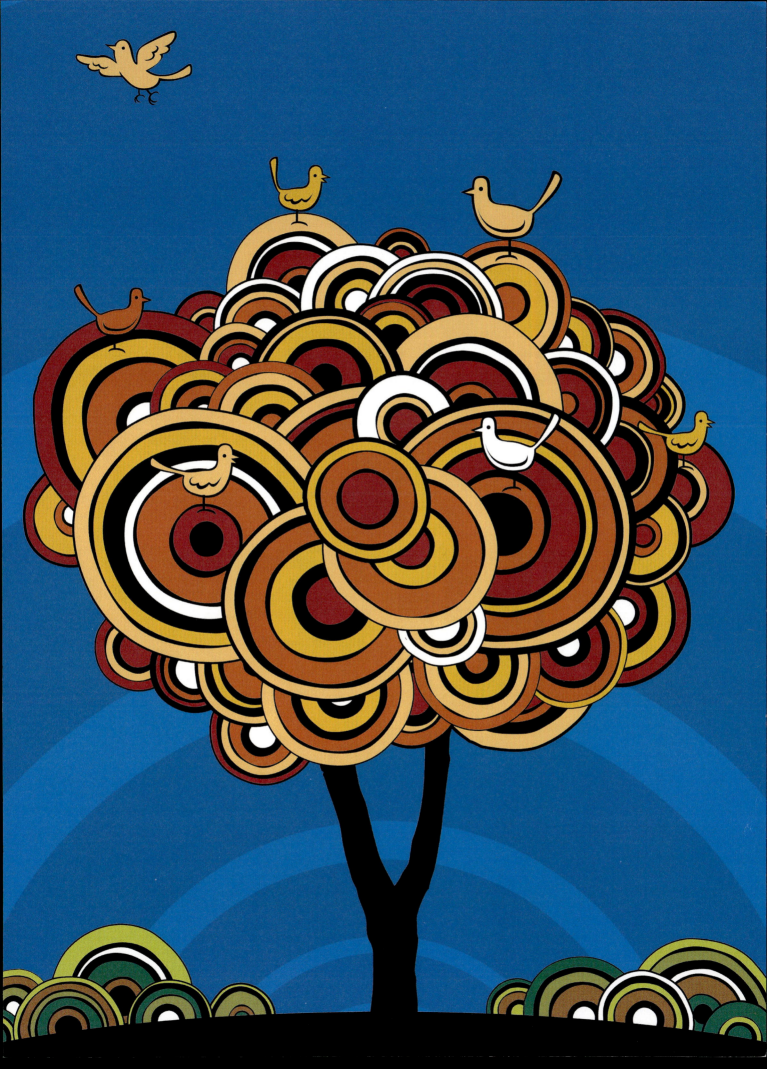

If I Could Fly

Imagine that you can fly.

Picture your wings.

What color are they?

What do they feel like?

Now imagine that you flap your wings and take off into the sky.

You can fly as high or as low as you want.

Look down and see all that is below you...

Can you see your house?

Your school?

Your favorite park and playground?

How far can you fly?

To another city?

To another state?

To another country?

To another planet?

To another galaxy?

Keep flying until you are ready to come home.

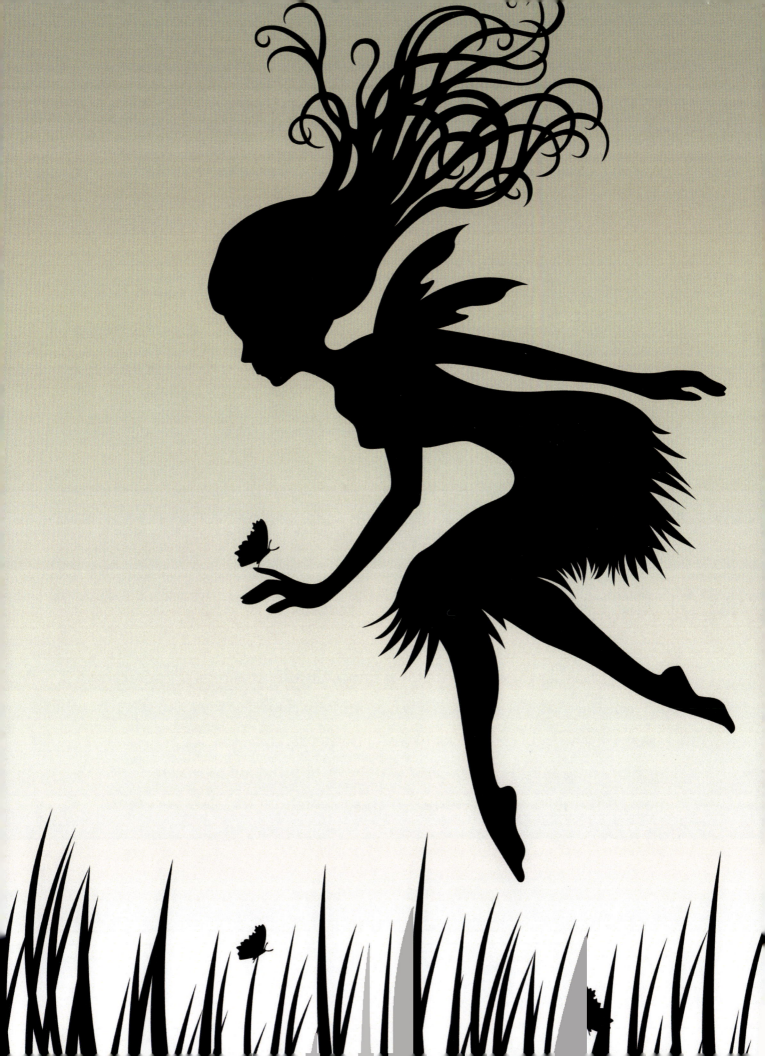

Clouds in the Sky

Imagine that you are lying in a huge field.

Take a deep breath and smell all the plants and grass that surround you.

Feel the softness of the grass on your feet, legs, back, arms, and head.

Wherever the grass touches, feel your body relax and settle into the ground.

Feel the weight of your body held by the Earth.

Above you is the sky, big and blue, with lots of floating clouds.

Wispy clouds.

Fluffy clouds.

Streaky clouds.

Polka-dotted clouds.

Clouds of different colors.

Pick a cloud and watch it as it slowly moves.

As it floats across the sky, watch it become different shapes and patterns.

Find another cloud and watch it move and change.

Here comes a cloud that looks like a giant heart.

Think of something you love and watch the cloud change into it.

Enjoy just lying here, relaxed in the grass, watching the clouds in the sky drift by.

A Trip in Your Spaceship

Imagine that you are blasting off into space.

See yourself putting on your spacesuit and helmet.

Go to your spaceship and get in.

Be sure to buckle your seatbelt!

Ten, nine, eight, seven, six, five, four, three, two, one…

Blast off!

Your spaceship takes off and goes up into the sky.

It gets higher and higher and higher…

Until you can see the whole earth from above.

Can you see the moon?

The stars?

Do you see any other planets?

Can you see the sun?

A comet?

Can you see your house?

The windows of your room?

Take as much time as you'd like flying through space in your spaceship.

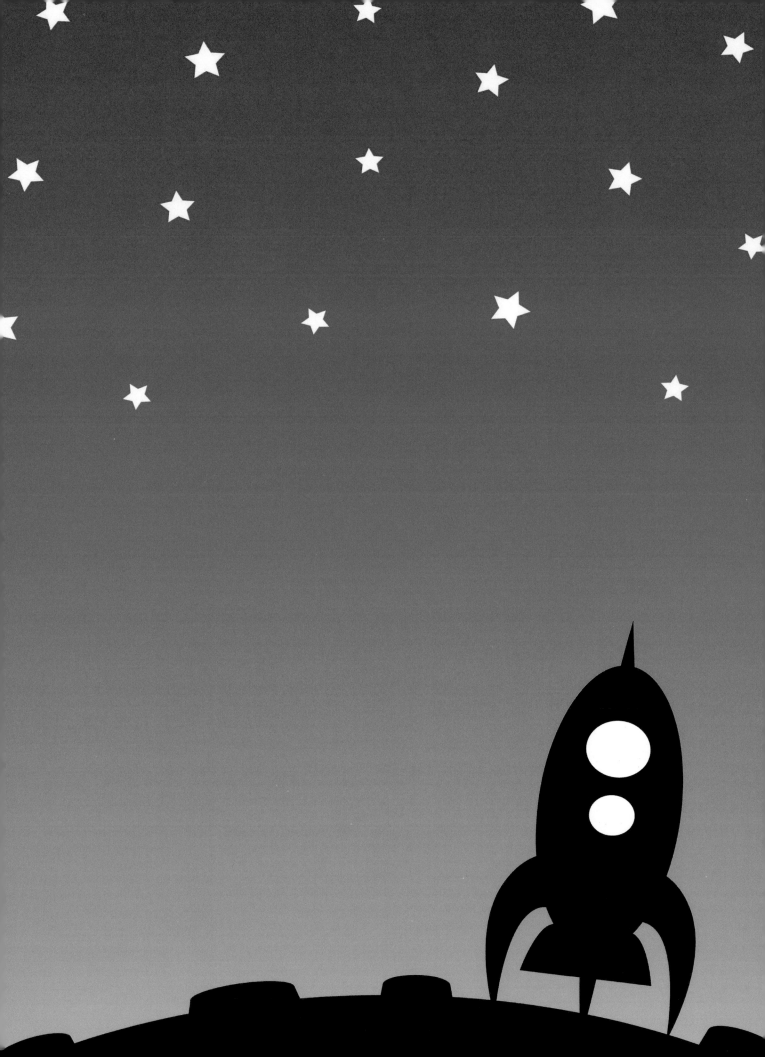

Enchanted Forest

Imagine that you are walking into a magical, enchanted forest.

You feel very safe while you are in this forest.

Look at the trees as you walk past them.

Do you see them smiling at you and making silly faces?

Take a deep breath and see if you smell anything magical in this forest.

Notice if you hear any sounds, like birds or the wind in the trees.

As you walk deeper into the forest, you feel your body shrinking.

Feeling very safe, you get smaller and smaller.

Up ahead you see some very magical creatures—

Gnomes and fairies!

They are friendly and the same size as you.

Follow them in the forest and see where they take you.

You are so small that you can go anywhere!

You can float on a leaf on the lake.

You can climb up a plant and into the petals of a flower.

You can even sit on the top of a mushroom.

Imagine all the places that you can explore in this enchanted forest.

Keep exploring with your new friends until you are ready to say goodbye.

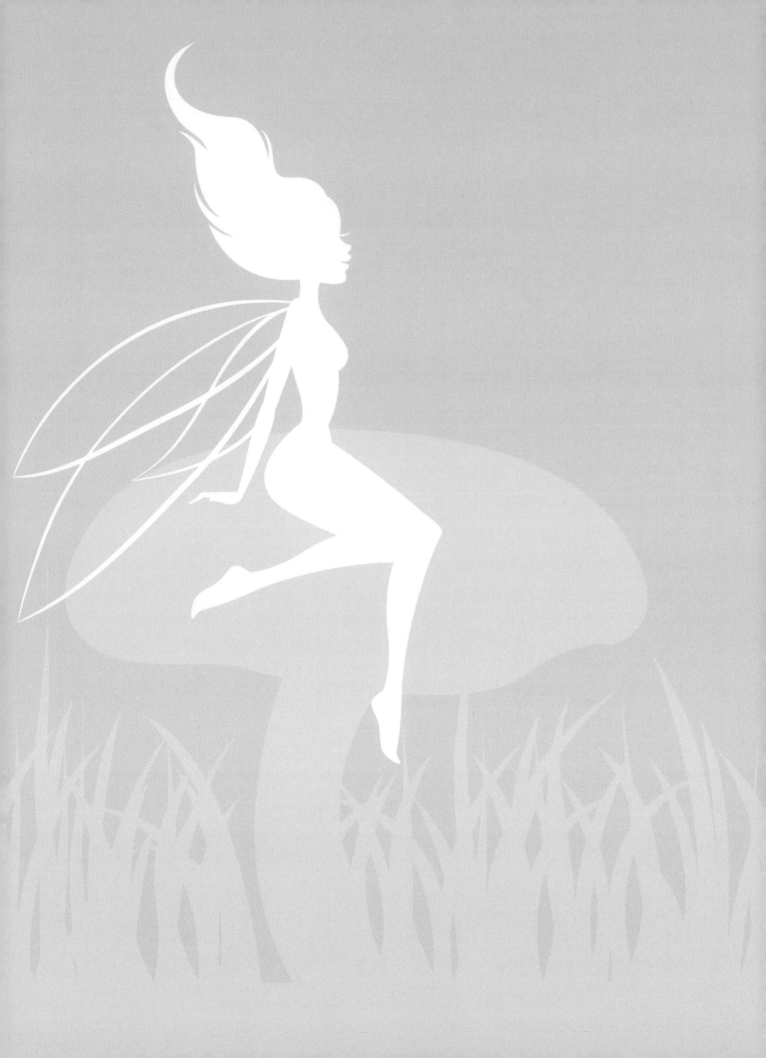

Take a Hike

Imagine that you are going on a hike anywhere in the world.

Picture where you are—

On a mountain?

Along the beach?

In a forest?

Next to a river?

Or even in your backyard.

As you walk, listen to the sound of your feet on the ground.

Feel the warmth of the sun…

The coolness of the breeze on your skin.

Do you hear or see any animals?

Take in a deep breath—

What do you smell?

Do you taste anything?

Enjoy the fresh air…

The blue sky…

And, when you are finished exploring, hike home.

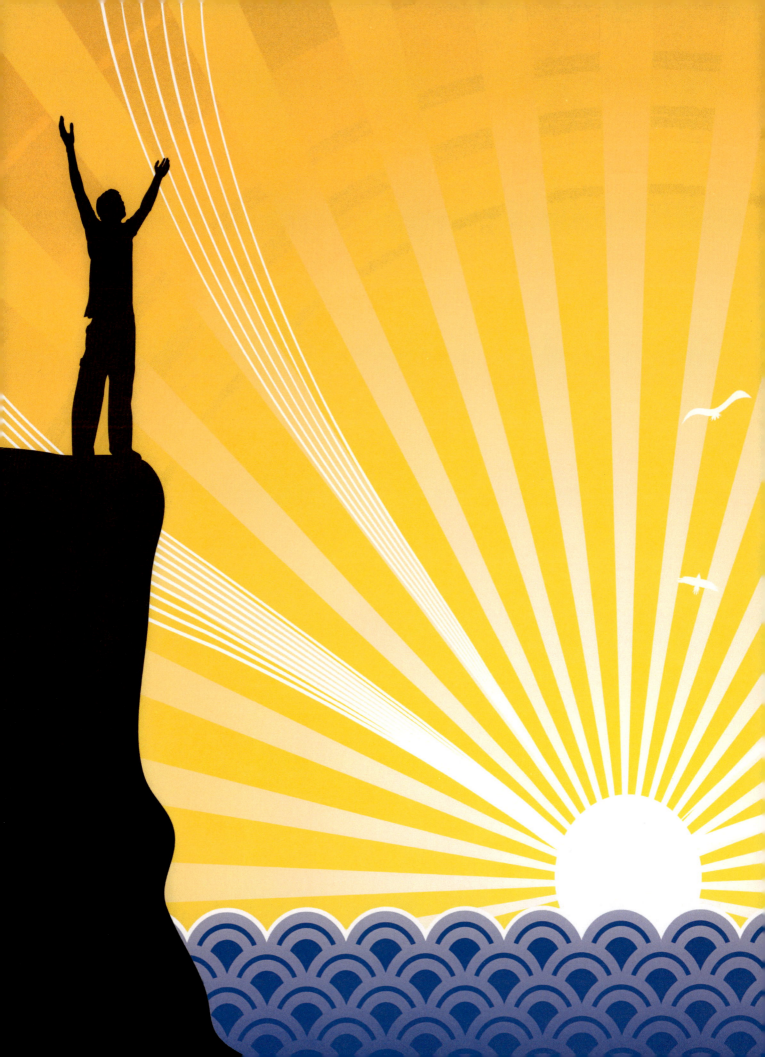

The Love Balloon

Imagine you have the biggest balloon in the world.

It can be any color you'd like.

Now imagine that you want to give this balloon to someone you love.

Take a deep breath in.

Now blow out imagining that you are filling the balloon with love.

Breathe in…

Breathe out…

Breathe in…

Breathe out…

Keep breathing in and out, filling up your balloon.

Tie a string around the bottom when it is full.

Hold onto the string, and feel this giant balloon lift you from the ground.

The balloon is so big that it can fly you anywhere in the world.

Imagine that the balloon carries you to this person that you love.

Give the balloon to them,

And feel how happy they are to receive this gift of love.

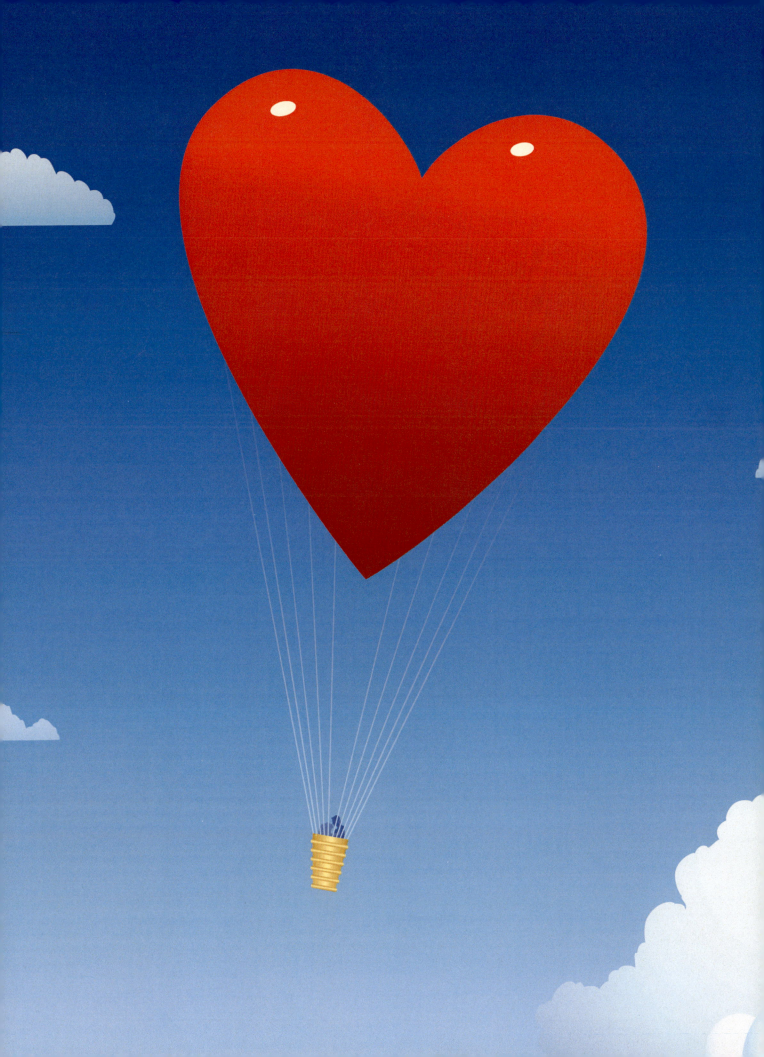

Under the Sea

Imagine that you are swimming under the ocean.

You have a little air tank, so you can stay under and breathe as long as you'd like.

Listen to the sound of your breath and let the sound relax you.

Does your breath sound like the sound of the ocean?

Feel how light your body is as it floats in the water.

Imagine that you swim to a place filled with all your favorite sea creatures.

Maybe you see whales…

Dolphins…

Seahorses…

Schools of colorful fish…

Rays…

Lobsters…

Sea turtles…

Any of your favorite sea animals… Picture them now…

Do you hear any sounds?

Whales singing?

The sound of waves above you?

Can you feel anything?

The water?

Seaweed tickling your toes?

The smooth skin of a dolphin?

Enjoy everything around you under the sea.

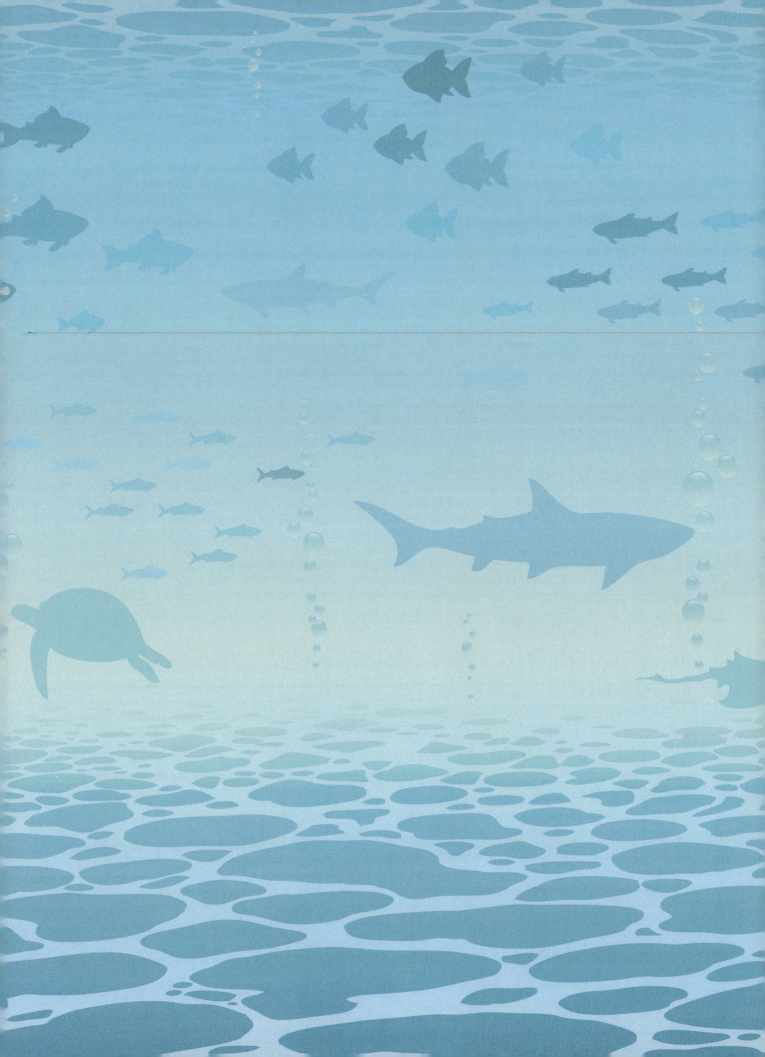

My Tree House

Imagine the most beautiful tree in the world.

Is it a palm tree?

An oak tree?

A tall tree?

A short tree?

Now imagine that you build a tree house in it.

Use all the tools you need to create your very own place in this tree.

Climb up into your tree house.

You can bring anything special with you (maybe a blanket or a stuffed animal).

Now imagine what you can see from your tree house.

An ocean view?

A forest full of trees?

Is it so high up that you can see all the way to a city far away?

Can you touch the sky?

Now imagine that you lie down in your tree house.

Can you hear the wind in the leaves of your tree?

Feel how safe your tree house makes you feel.

Nothing can hurt you when you are in your tree house.

You can come back to your tree house anytime you'd like, you just have to close your eyes.

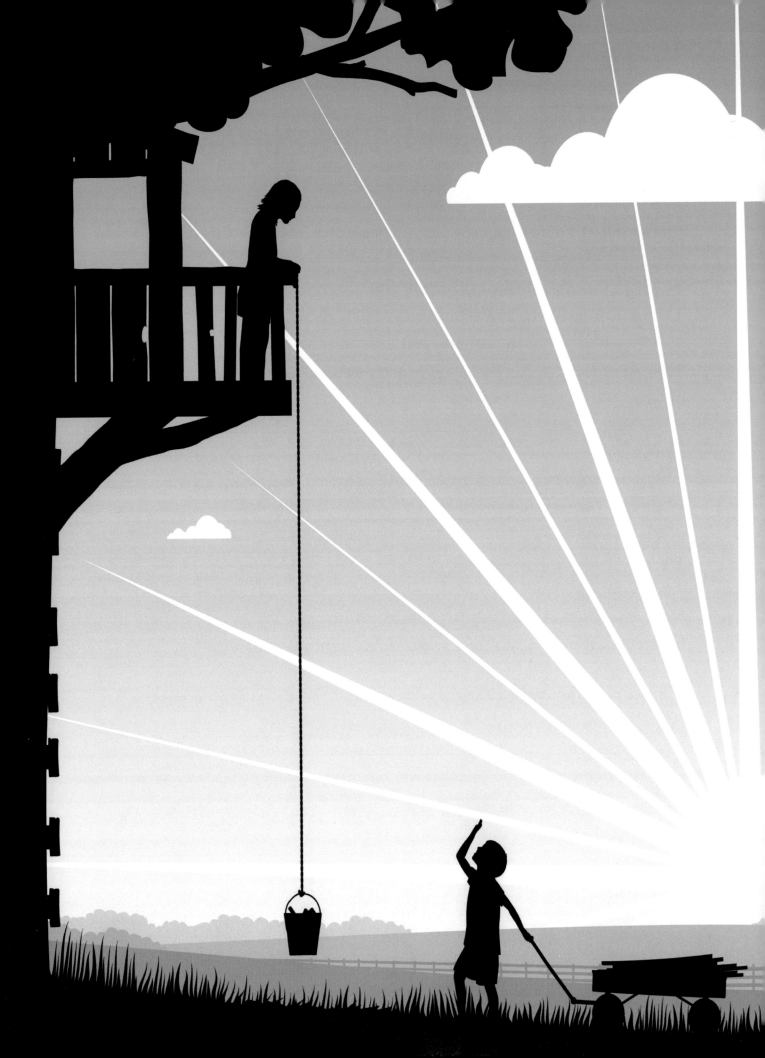

Magic Flower Potion

Imagine that you are mixing a magic potion.
In front of you is a huge pot.
Put anything you'd like in the pot.
Maybe some strawberries, glitter, and a bird feather…
Maybe a marble, a toy car, and a shark's tooth.
Now imagine that the potion starts to boil and bubble.
Stir it…
And stir it…
And stir it….
Scoop out some potion and take a little sip.
What does your magic potion do?
Is it a love potion?
A peace potion?
A silly potion?
Now imagine that the potion changes color.
It becomes a potion that turns your breath into flowers.
Take a sip.
Can you see them when you exhale?
Imagine that your potion changes color again.
It's a relaxation potion now.
Imagine you take a sip.
Feel how it relaxes your feet…
Your legs…
Your belly…
Your arms…
Your back…
Your head and face…
Until your whole body feels completely relaxed.

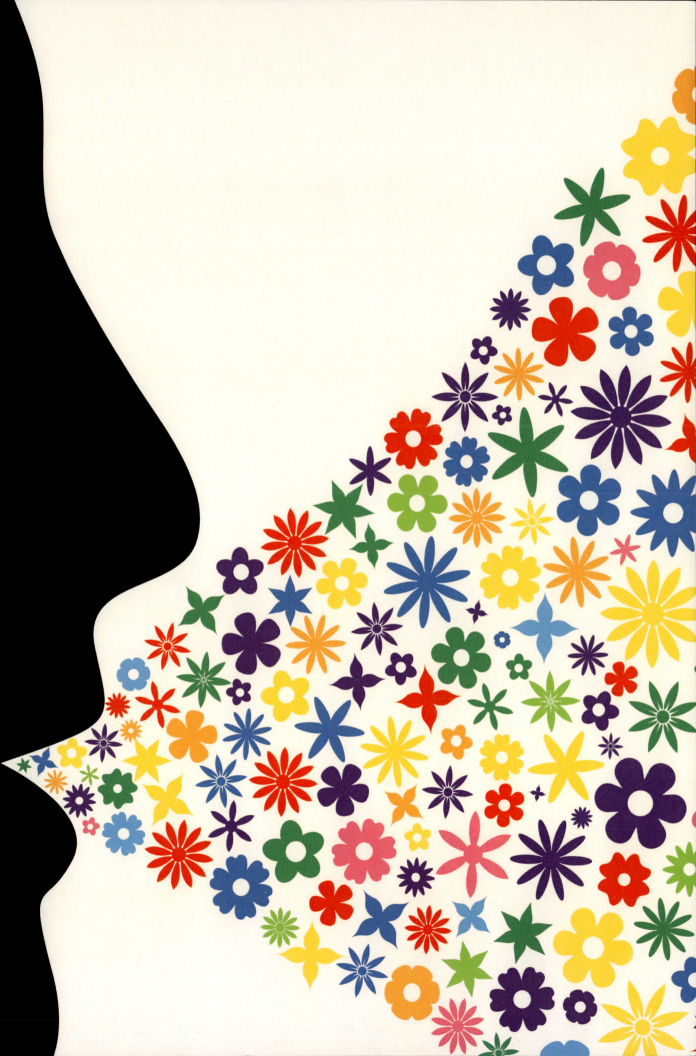

Planting a Seed

Imagine that you have a magical seed in your hands.

Whisper a secret to the seed.

Tell it what you'd like it to grow into.

Now dig a hole in the ground.

Plant your seed in the hole and cover it with dirt.

Imagine that it starts to rain.

Water slowly soaks into the soil.

Now the sun comes out and shines brightly on the garden.

You start to see a tiny sprout poke up out of the soil.

Tangled roots grow down into the ground.

And the seed grows

And grows…

And grows…

What has it become?

A tree?

A flower?

A strawberry plant?

A magical fairy tree?

Enjoy this beautiful thing your seed has grown into.

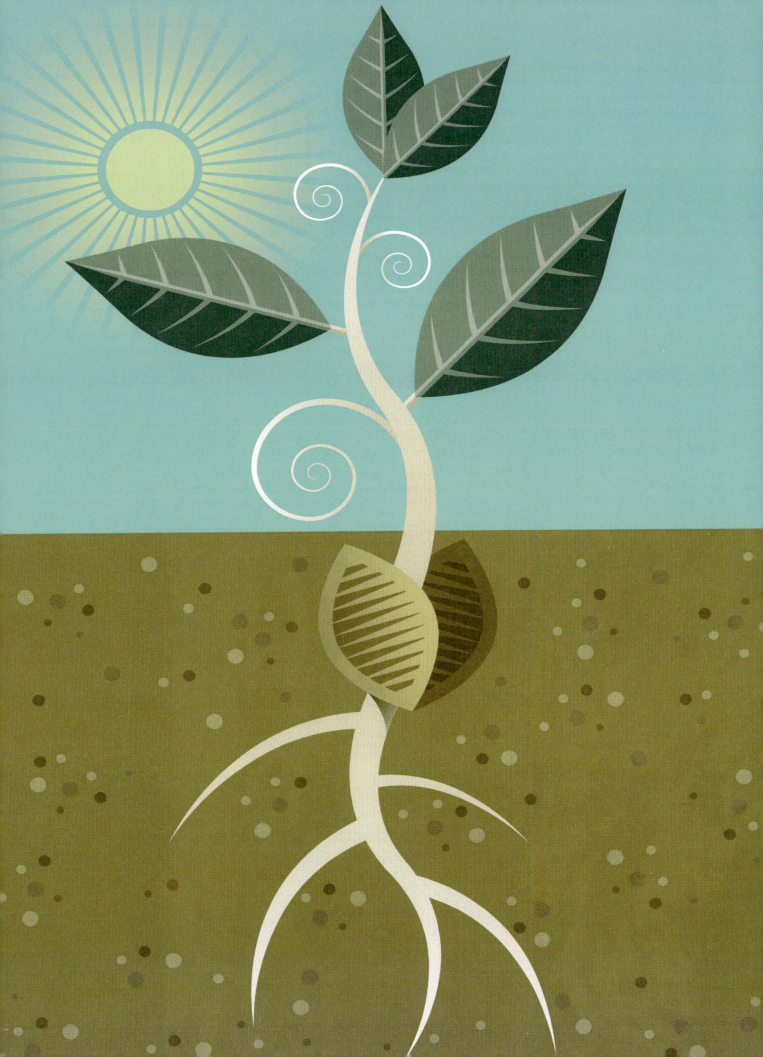

Finger Lights

Choose a color.

Rosy red?

Bright orange?

Sunshine yellow?

Leaf green?

Sky blue?

Pretty purple?

Now see your toes light up in your favorite color.

When your toes turn this color, feel your toes relax.

Now see your legs light up,

And your legs relax.

Your belly lights up,

And your belly relaxes.

Your back lights up,

And your back relaxes.

Your head and face light up,

And they relax, too.

Now see the colorful light move down your arms.

And your arms relax, too.

Your whole body is filled with light,

So much light that this light starts to shoot out of the tips of your fingers.

You can draw in the air with your "finger lights."

You can send some of this colorful, relaxing light to your family…

To your friends…

You can even send light around the world to people you don't know.

Now feel your whole body relaxed and bright.

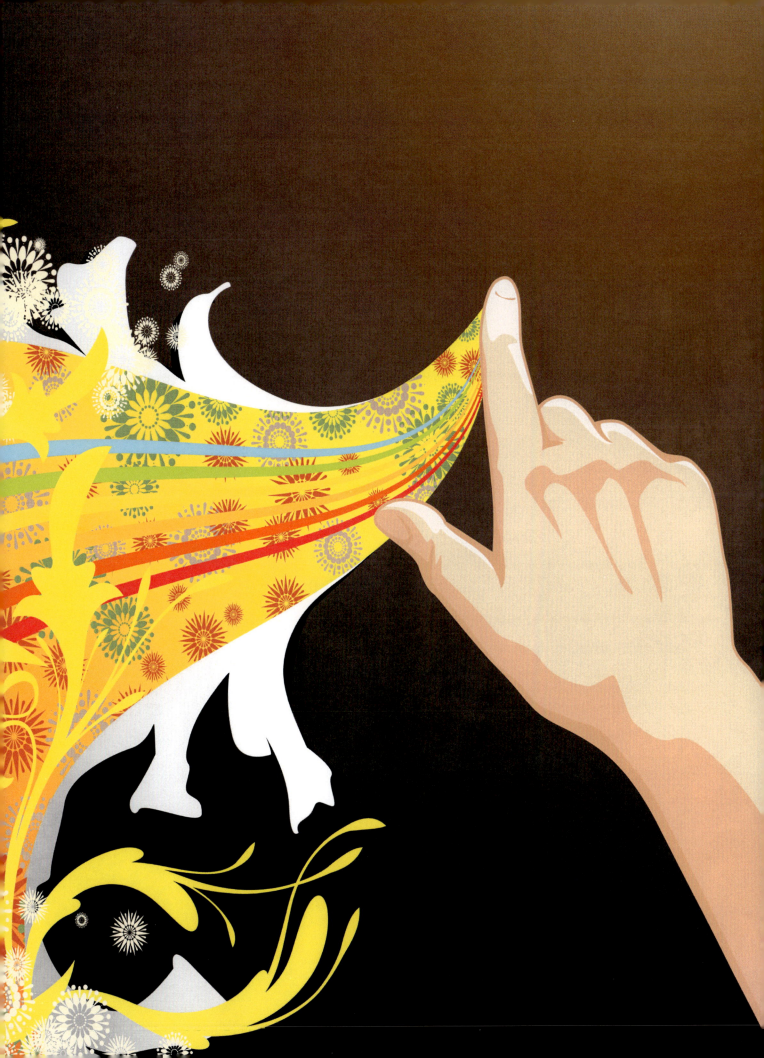

Loving Kindness

Imagine that you are sending love to yourself.

How would you do this?

Would you mail yourself a valentine?

Would you use your voice?

Would you give yourself a hug?

Would you blow yourself a kiss?

Now tell each part of your body that you love it:

I love you, feet.

I love you, legs.

I love you, belly.

I love you, back.

I love you, arms.

I love you, face.

Notice how your body feels when you tell it that you love it.

Now think of someone you love very much.

Maybe someone in your family or your best friend.

Send them some love.

Now think of someone who is mean or unfriendly.

Send this person some love, too.

Sometimes people are mean because they don't feel loved.

So send this person some extra love.

Now think of all the people all over the world.

Send them some love, too.

Now imagine all of these people you sent love to…

And now imagine that all of those people send love back to you.

You might even be able to feel it!

Additional Information

Visit ImaginationsForKids.com for additional resources, activities, and information about relaxation for children.

This book is available at quantity discounts with bulk purchase for educational, business, or promotional use. We are also available for special events, workshops, and classes.

For information, please contact:
Web: ImaginationsForKids.com
Email: info@imaginationsforkids.com

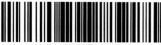

Made in the USA
Lexington, KY
22 November 2017